MW01516484

THIS JOURNAL BELONGS TO

_____

_____

date ....

DAYS SOBER

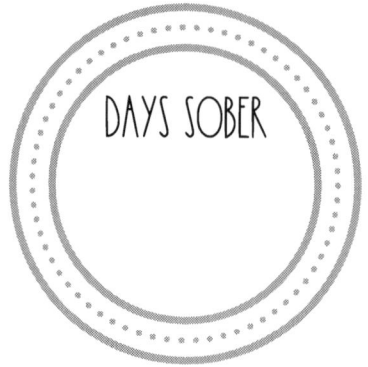

> It does not matter how slowly you go as long as you do not stop. — Confucius

TODAY I FEEL ....

TODAY I'M GRATEFUL FOR

1.

2.

3.

TODAY MY GOALS ARE

....

....

....

my mood today:

(1) (2) (3) (4) (5) (6) (7) (8) (9) (10)

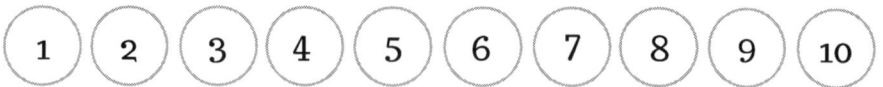

today i will support
MY SOBRIETY
by doing
this ONE thing

thoughts about today:

date

...

DAYS SOBER

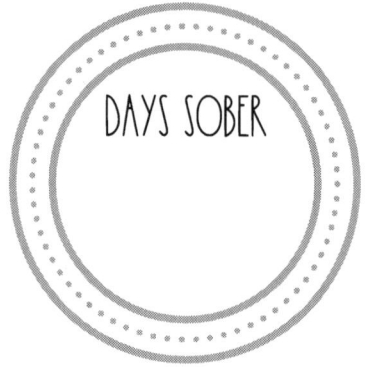

> "The goal isn't to be sober. The goal is to love yourself so much that you don't need to drink."
>
> Unknown

TODAY I FEEL

...

TODAY I'M GRATEFUL FOR

1.

2.

3.

TODAY MY GOALS ARE

...

...

...

my mood today:

(1) (2) (3) (4) (5) (6) (7) (8) (9) (10)

today i will support MY SOBRIETY by doing this ONE thing:

thoughts about today:

date ....

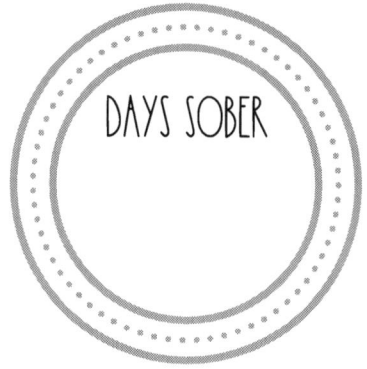

DAYS SOBER

> Recovery is an acceptance that your life is in shambles and you have to change. **J.L. Curtis**

TODAY I FEEL ....

TODAY I'M GRATEFUL FOR

1.

2.

3.

TODAY MY GOALS ARE

....

....

....

my mood today:

(1) (2) (3) (4) (5) (6) (7) (8) (9) (10)

today i will support MY SOBRIETY *by doing* this ONE thing

thoughts about today:

date ....

DAYS SOBER

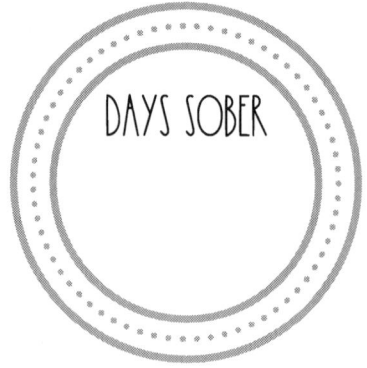

"Recovery is about progression not perfection. Unknown"

TODAY I FEEL ....

TODAY I'M GRATEFUL FOR

1.

2.

3.

TODAY MY GOALS ARE

....

....

....

my mood today:

(1) (2) (3) (4) (5) (6) (7) (8) (9) (10)

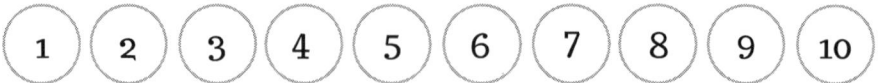

today i will support MY SOBRIETY *by doing* this ONE thing:

thoughts about today:

date ....

DAYS SOBER

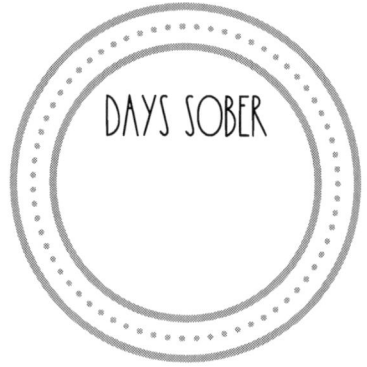

> Recovery didn't open the gates of heaven and let me in. Recovery opened the gates of hell and let me out! Unknown

TODAY I FEEL ....

TODAY I'M GRATEFUL FOR

1.

2.

3.

TODAY MY GOALS ARE

....

....

....

my mood today:

(1) (2) (3) (4) (5) (6) (7) (8) (9) (10)

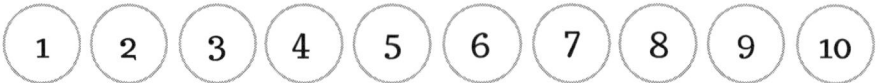

today i will support MY SOBRIETY *by doing* this ONE thing

thoughts about today:

date ....

DAYS SOBER

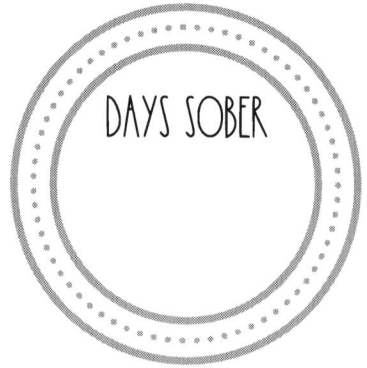

," Believe you can
and you're
halfway there. Th. Roosevelt
"

TODAY I FEEL ....

TODAY I'M GRATEFUL FOR

1.

2.

3.

TODAY MY GOALS ARE

....

....

....

my mood today:

(1) (2) (3) (4) (5) (6) (7) (8) (9) (10)

today i will support
MY SOBRIETY
by doing
this ONE thing.

thoughts about today:

date

_____

DAYS SOBER

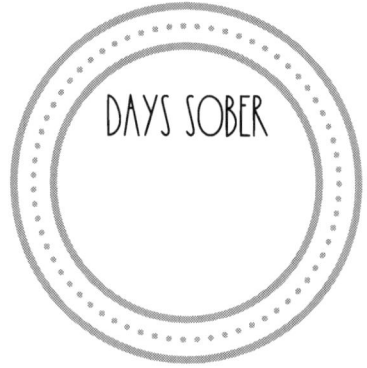

> The best time to plant a tree was 20 years ago. The second best time is now. — Chinese Proverb

TODAY I FEEL

_____

TODAY I'M GRATEFUL FOR

1.

2.

3.

TODAY MY GOALS ARE

_____

_____

_____

my mood today:

(1) (2) (3) (4) (5) (6) (7) (8) (9) (10)

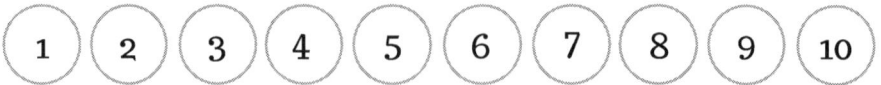

today i will support MY SOBRIETY by doing this ONE thing:

thoughts about today:

date ....

"

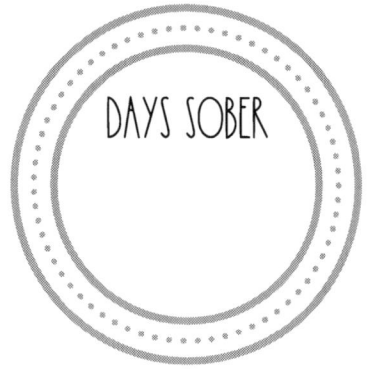

The most
common way
people give up
their power is by
thinking that
they don't
have any.   A. Walker

"

TODAY I FEEL ....

TODAY I'M GRATEFUL FOR

1.

2.

3.

TODAY MY GOALS ARE

....

....

....

my mood today:

(1) (2) (3) (4) (5) (6) (7) (8) (9) (10)

today i will support
MY SOBRIETY
by doing
this ONE thing:

thoughts about today:

date ....

DAYS SOBER

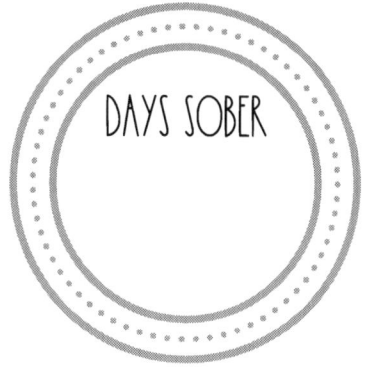

" The only person
you are destined
to become is the
person you
decide to be. R.W. Emerson

TODAY I FEEL ....

TODAY I'M GRATEFUL FOR

1.

2.

3.

TODAY MY GOALS ARE

....

....

....

my mood today:

(1) (2) (3) (4) (5) (6) (7) (8) (9) (10)

today i will support
MY SOBRIETY
by doing
this ONE thing

thoughts about today:

date

_____

DAYS SOBER

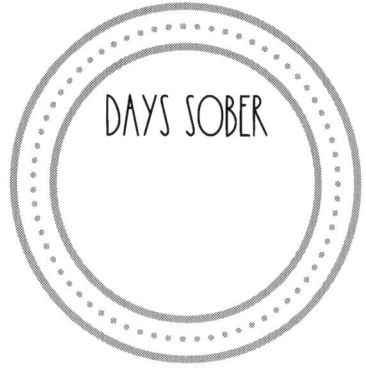

> I am not defined
> by my relapses,
> but by my
> decision to remain
> in recovery
> despite them. Unknown

TODAY I FEEL

....

TODAY I'M GRATEFUL FOR

1.

2.

3.

TODAY MY GOALS ARE

....

....

....

my mood today:

(1) (2) (3) (4) (5) (6) (7) (8) (9) (10)

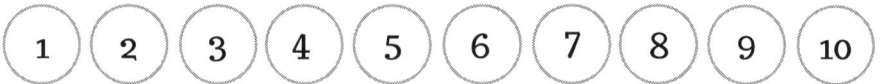

today i will support
MY SOBRIETY
by doing
this ONE thing

thoughts about today:

date ....

DAYS SOBER

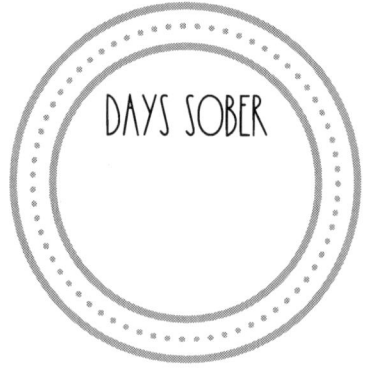

66 The best way out is always through." R. Frost 99

TODAY I FEEL ....

TODAY I'M GRATEFUL FOR

1.

2.

3.

TODAY MY GOALS ARE

....

....

....

my mood today:

(1) (2) (3) (4) (5) (6) (7) (8) (9) (10)

today i will support MY SOBRIETY *by doing* this ONE thing

thoughts about today:

date ....

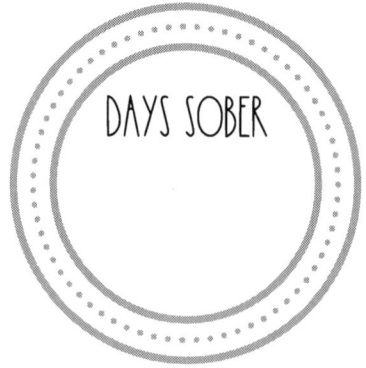

DAYS SOBER

" Fall seven times,
stand up eight.
Japanese Proverb "

TODAY I FEEL ....

TODAY I'M GRATEFUL FOR

1.

2.

3.

TODAY MY GOALS ARE

....

....

....

my mood today:

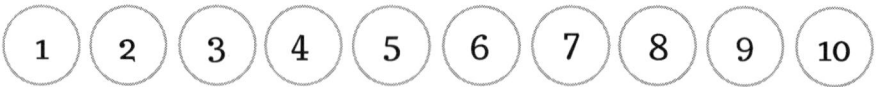

① 1 ② 2 ③ 3 ④ 4 ⑤ 5 ⑥ 6 ⑦ 7 ⑧ 8 ⑨ 9 ⑩ 10

today i will support
MY SOBRIETY
by doing
this ONE thing:

thoughts about today:

date ....

DAYS SOBER

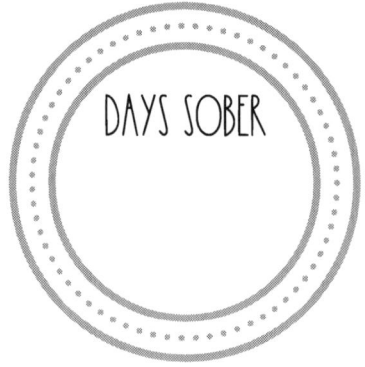

"
You may have to
fight a battle
more than once
to win it. M. Thatcher
"

TODAY I FEEL ....

TODAY I'M GRATEFUL FOR

1.

2.

3.

TODAY MY GOALS ARE

....

....

....

my mood today:

(1) (2) (3) (4) (5) (6) (7) (8) (9) (10)

today i will support
MY SOBRIETY
by doing
this ONE thing:

thoughts about today:

date ....

DAYS SOBER

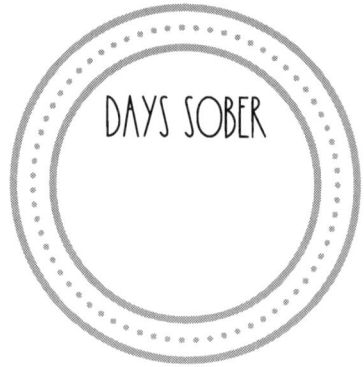

> Every worth
> act is difficult.
> Ascent is always
> difficult. Descent
> is easy and
> often slippery.　M. Gandhi

TODAY I FEEL ....

TODAY I'M GRATEFUL FOR

1.

2.

3.

TODAY MY GOALS ARE

....

....

....

my mood today:

(1) (2) (3) (4) (5) (6) (7) (8) (9) (10)

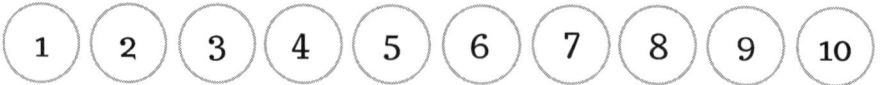

today i will support
MY SOBRIETY
by doing
this ONE thing:

thoughts about today:

date

....

DAYS SOBER

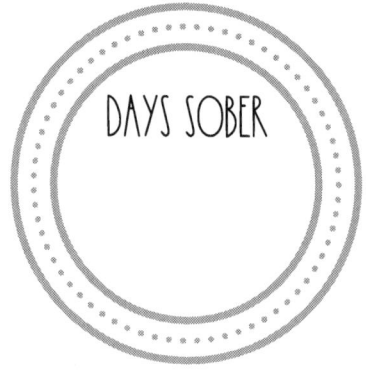

> **Success is the sum of small efforts, repeated day in and day out.** R. Collier

TODAY I FEEL

....

TODAY I'M GRATEFUL FOR

1.

2.

3.

TODAY MY GOALS ARE

....

....

....

my mood today:

(1) (2) (3) (4) (5) (6) (7) (8) (9) (10)

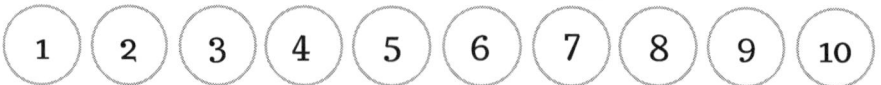

today i will support MY SOBRIETY by doing this ONE thing:

thoughts about today:

date ....

DAYS SOBER

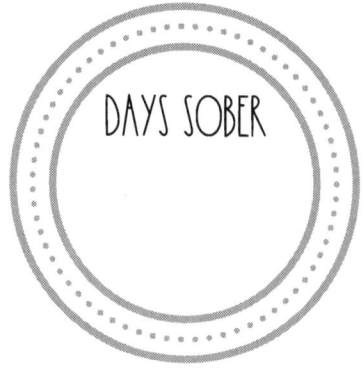

Nothing is
impossible; the
word itself says,
'I'm possible!' A. Hepburn

TODAY I FEEL ....

TODAY I'M GRATEFUL FOR

1.

2.

3.

TODAY MY GOALS ARE

....

....

....

my mood today:

(1) (2) (3) (4) (5) (6) (7) (8) (9) (10)

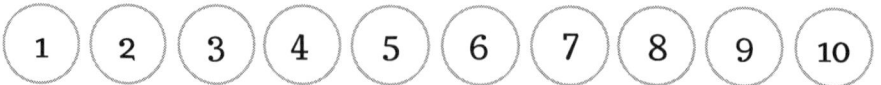

today i will support
MY SOBRIETY
by doing
this ONE thing:

thoughts about today:

date ....

DAYS SOBER

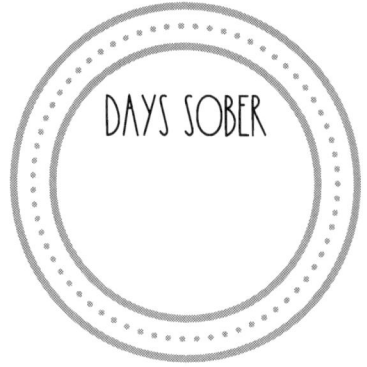

> " Only through experience of trial and suffering can the soul be strengthened, ambition inspired, and success achieved.   H. Keller

TODAY I FEEL ....

TODAY I'M GRATEFUL FOR

1.

2.

3.

TODAY MY GOALS ARE

....

....

....

my mood today:

1   2   3   4   5   6   7   8   9   10

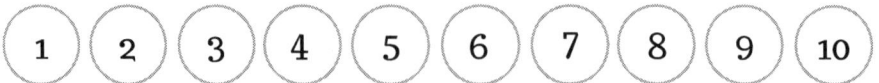

today i will support
MY SOBRIETY
by doing
this ONE thing:

thoughts about today:

date

....

DAYS SOBER

66 99

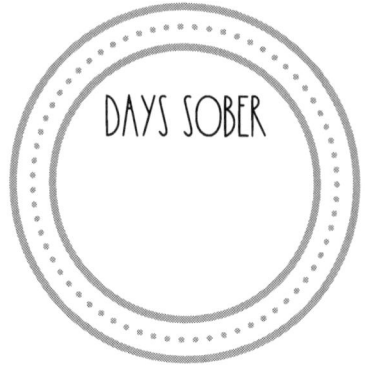

"Whether you think you can or you think you can't, you're right." H. Ford

TODAY I FEEL

....

TODAY I'M GRATEFUL FOR

1.

2.

3.

TODAY MY GOALS ARE

....

....

....

my mood today:

(1) (2) (3) (4) (5) (6) (7) (8) (9) (10)

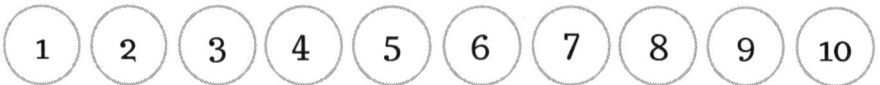

today i will support
MY SOBRIETY
by doing
this ONE thing:

thoughts about today:

date ....

DAYS SOBER

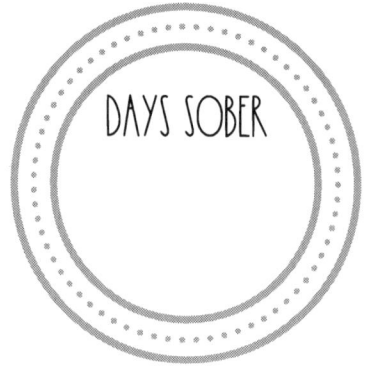

" Though no one can go back and make a brand new start, anyone can start from now and make a brand new ending. " C. Bard

TODAY I FEEL ....

TODAY I'M GRATEFUL FOR

1.

2.

3.

TODAY MY GOALS ARE

....

....

....

my mood today:

(1) (2) (3) (4) (5) (6) (7) (8) (9) (10)

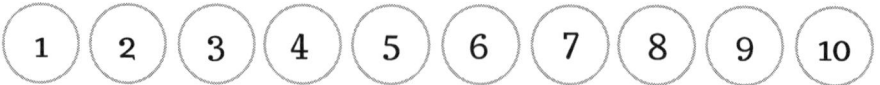

today i will support MY SOBRIETY by doing this ONE thing

thoughts about today:

date ....

DAYS SOBER

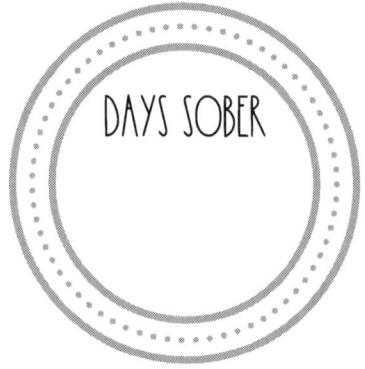

"
It always seems
impossible
until it's done. N. Mandela
"

TODAY I FEEL ....

TODAY I'M GRATEFUL FOR

1.

2.

3.

TODAY MY GOALS ARE

....

....

....

my mood today:

(1) (2) (3) (4) (5) (6) (7) (8) (9) (10)

today i will support
MY SOBRIETY
by doing
this ONE thing:

thoughts about today:

date ....

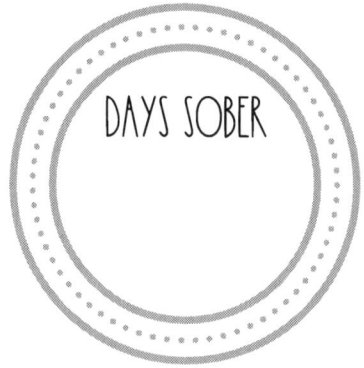

" When everything
seems to be going
against you,
remember that
the airplane takes
off against the
wind, not with it.   H. Ford "

TODAY I FEEL ....

TODAY I'M GRATEFUL FOR

1.

2.

3.

TODAY MY GOALS ARE

....

....

....

my mood today:

(1) (2) (3) (4) (5) (6) (7) (8) (9) (10)

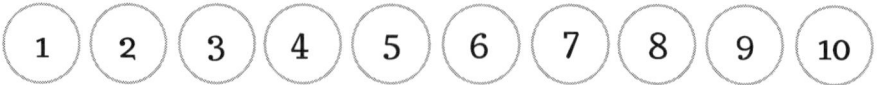

today i will support
MY SOBRIETY
by doing
this ONE thing

thoughts about today:

date ....

DAYS SOBER

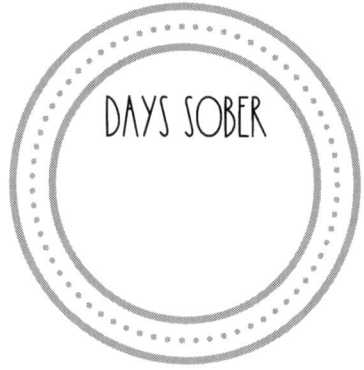

> **Every strike brings me closer to the next home run.** B. Ruth

TODAY I FEEL ....

TODAY I'M GRATEFUL FOR

1.

2.

3.

TODAY MY GOALS ARE

....

....

....

my mood today:

(1) (2) (3) (4) (5) (6) (7) (8) (9) (10)

today i will support
MY SOBRIETY
by doing
this ONE thing:

thoughts about today:

date ....

DAYS SOBER

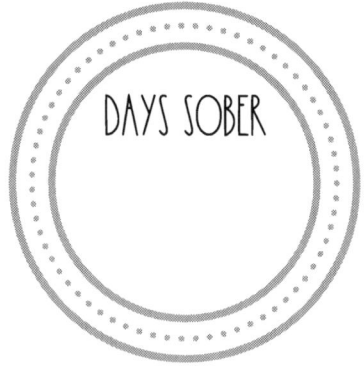

"
If you can quit
for a day, you
can quit for a
lifetime. B. A. Sáenz
"

TODAY I FEEL ....

TODAY I'M GRATEFUL FOR

1.

2.

3.

TODAY MY GOALS ARE

....

....

....

my mood today:

(1) (2) (3) (4) (5) (6) (7) (8) (9) (10)

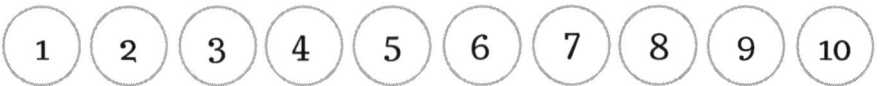

today i will support
MY SOBRIETY
by doing
this ONE thing

thoughts about today:

date ....

DAYS SOBER

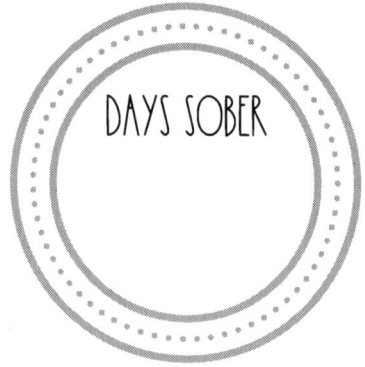

> There is no shame
> in beginning again,
> for you to get a
> chance to build
> bigger and better
> than before.   Unknown

TODAY I FEEL ....

TODAY I'M GRATEFUL FOR

1.

2.

3.

TODAY MY GOALS ARE

....

....

....

my mood today:

(1) (2) (3) (4) (5) (6) (7) (8) (9) (10)

today i will support
MY SOBRIETY
by doing
this ONE thing:

thoughts about today:

date ....

DAYS SOBER

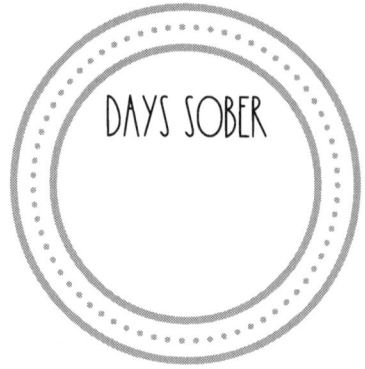

" There's not
a drug on earth
that can make
life meaningful.   Unknown "

TODAY I FEEL ....

TODAY I'M GRATEFUL FOR

1.

2.

3.

TODAY MY GOALS ARE

....

....

....

my mood today:

(1) (2) (3) (4) (5) (6) (7) (8) (9) (10)

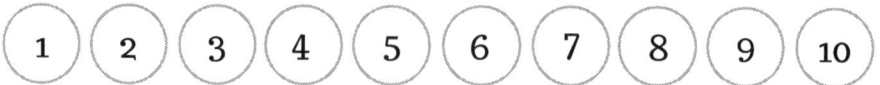

today i will support
MY SOBRIETY
by doing
this ONE thing.

thoughts about today:

date ....

DAYS SOBER

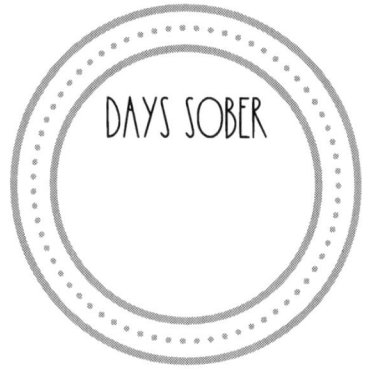

"
Be stronger than
your strongest
excuse.   Unknown
"

TODAY I FEEL ....

TODAY I'M GRATEFUL FOR

1.

2.

3.

TODAY MY GOALS ARE

....

....

....

my mood today:

(1) (2) (3) (4) (5) (6) (7) (8) (9) (10)

today i will support
MY SOBRIETY
by doing
this ONE thing:

thoughts about today:

date ....

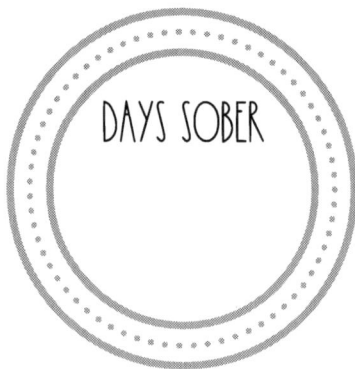

DAYS SOBER

"

It's a beautiful day
to be sober.   Unknown

"

TODAY I FEEL ....

TODAY I'M GRATEFUL FOR

1.

2.

3.

TODAY MY GOALS ARE

....

....

....

my mood today:

(1) (2) (3) (4) (5) (6) (7) (8) (9) (10)

today i will support
MY SOBRIETY
by doing
this ONE thing:

thoughts about today:

date ....

DAYS SOBER

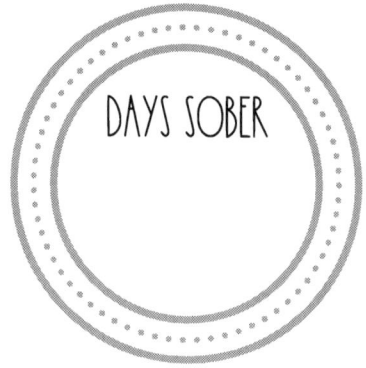

" It is often in the
darkest skies
that we see the
brightest stars. R. Evans "

TODAY I FEEL ....

TODAY I'M GRATEFUL FOR

1.

2.

3.

TODAY MY GOALS ARE

....

....

....

my mood today:

(1) (2) (3) (4) (5) (6) (7) (8) (9) (10)

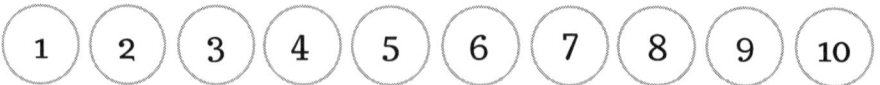

today i will support
MY SOBRIETY
by doing
this ONE thing

thoughts about today:

date ....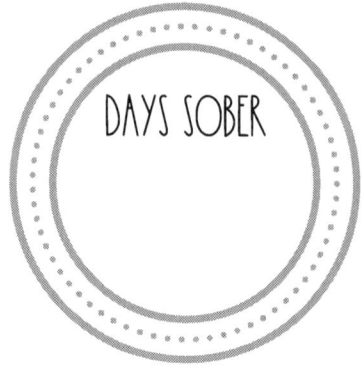

DAYS SOBER

"
Recovery is hard.
Regret is harder. B. Burgunder
"

TODAY I FEEL ....

TODAY I'M GRATEFUL FOR

1.

2.

3.

TODAY MY GOALS ARE

....

....

....

my mood today:

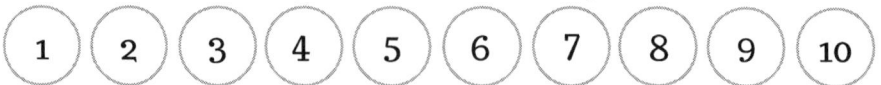

① 1 ② 2 ③ 3 ④ 4 ⑤ 5 ⑥ 6 ⑦ 7 ⑧ 8 ⑨ 9 ⑩ 10

today i will support
MY SOBRIETY
by doing
this ONE thing

thoughts about today:

date ....

DAYS SOBER

"

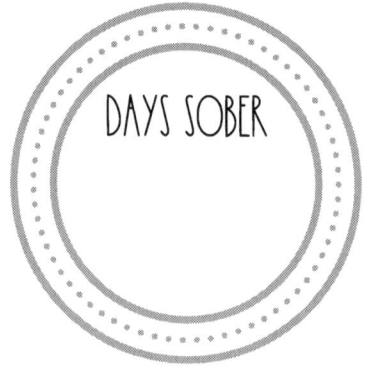

One small step is
worth more than a
thousand steps
planned.   Unknown

TODAY I FEEL ....

TODAY I'M GRATEFUL FOR

1.

2.

3.

TODAY MY GOALS ARE

....

....

....

my mood today:

(1) (2) (3) (4) (5) (6) (7) (8) (9) (10)

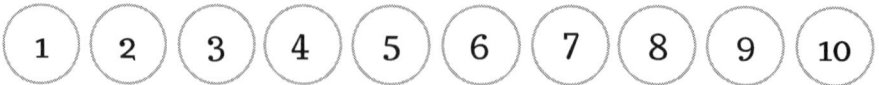

today i will support
MY SOBRIETY
by doing
this ONE thing:

thoughts about today:

_____

_____

_____

_____

_____

_____

_____

_____

_____

_____

date ....

DAYS SOBER

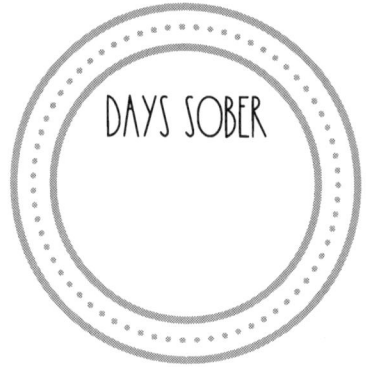

> Courage isn't having the strength to go on – it is going on when you don't have strength.   N. Bonaparte

TODAY I FEEL ....

TODAY I'M GRATEFUL FOR

1.
2.
3.

TODAY MY GOALS ARE

....

....

....

my mood today:

(1) (2) (3) (4) (5) (6) (7) (8) (9) (10)

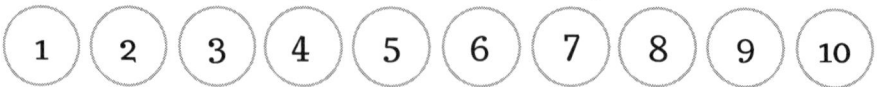

today i will support
MY SOBRIETY
by doing
this ONE thing:

thoughts about today:

MY MONTH *at a glance*

HABIT TRACKER

MONTH: _____

COLOR   ESSENTIAL HABITS

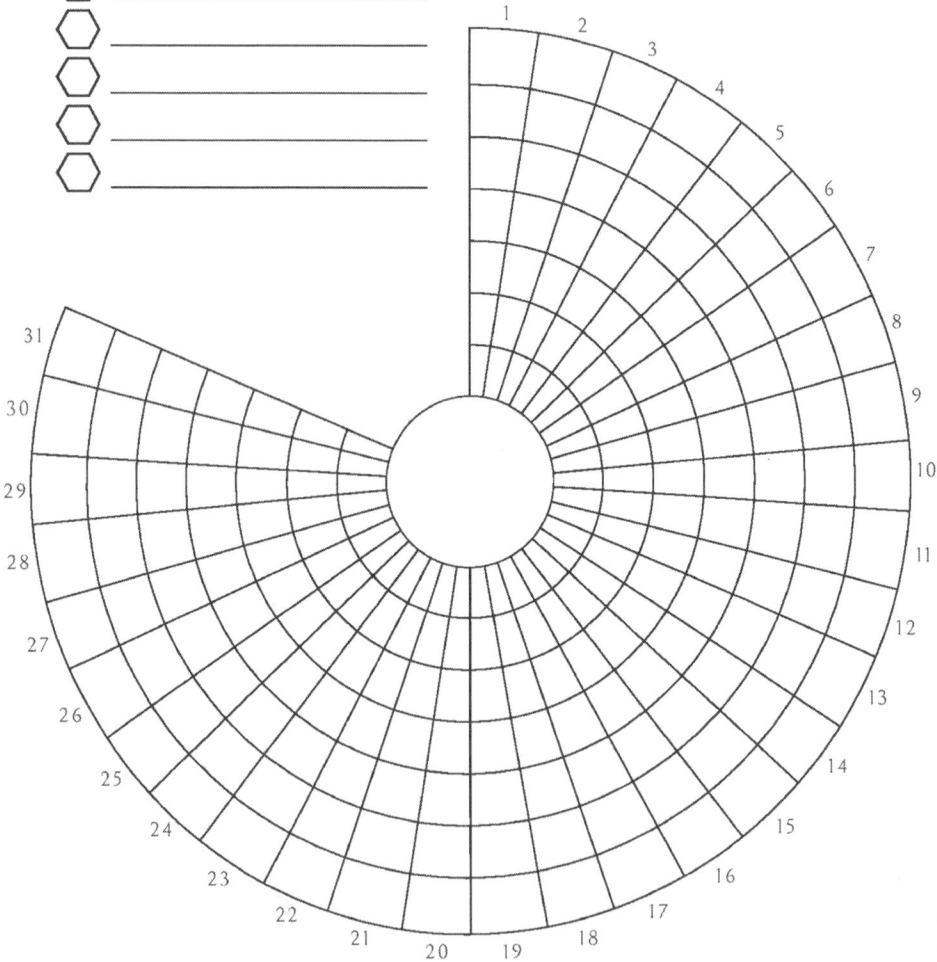

⬡ _____

⬡ _____

⬡ _____

⬡ _____

⬡ _____

⬡ _____

⬡ _____

date ....

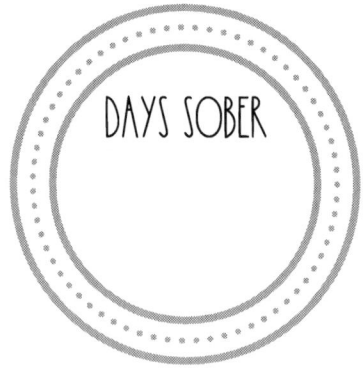

DAYS SOBER

" Don't let the past
steal your
present. T. Guillemets "

TODAY I FEEL ....

TODAY I'M GRATEFUL FOR

1.

2.

3.

TODAY MY GOALS ARE

....

....

....

my mood today:

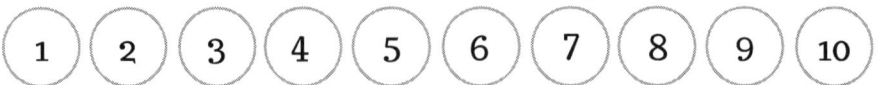

today i will support
MY SOBRIETY
by doing
this ONE thing:

thoughts about today:

date ....

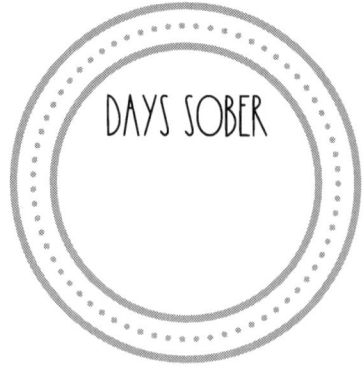

DAYS SOBER

He conquers
who endures. Persius

TODAY I FEEL ....

TODAY I'M GRATEFUL FOR

1.

2.

3.

TODAY MY GOALS ARE

....

....

....

my mood today:

(1) (2) (3) (4) (5) (6) (7) (8) (9) (10)

today i will support
MY SOBRIETY
by doing
this ONE thing:

thoughts about today:

date ....

DAYS SOBER

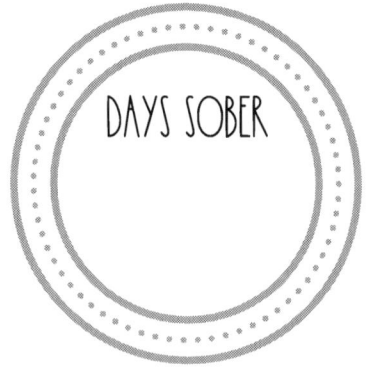

" Great acts are
made up of small
deeds. Lao Tzu "

TODAY I FEEL ....

TODAY I'M GRATEFUL FOR

1.

2.

3.

TODAY MY GOALS ARE

....

....

....

my mood today:

(1) (2) (3) (4) (5) (6) (7) (8) (9) (10)

today i will support
MY SOBRIETY
by doing
this ONE thing:

thoughts about today:

date _____

DAYS SOBER

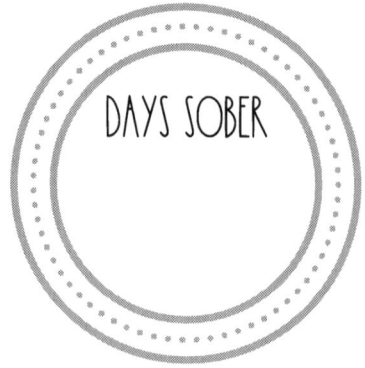

> Experience is not
> what happens to
> you, it is what you
> do with what
> happens to you. A. Huxley

TODAY I FEEL _____

TODAY I'M GRATEFUL FOR

1.

2.

3.

TODAY MY GOALS ARE

_____

_____

_____

my mood today:

(1) (2) (3) (4) (5) (6) (7) (8) (9) (10)

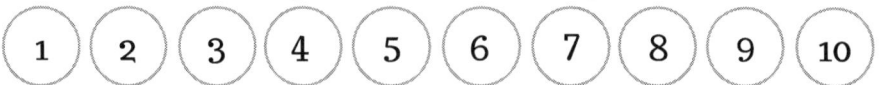

today i will support
MY SOBRIETY
by doing
this ONE thing:

thoughts about today:

date ....

DAYS SOBER

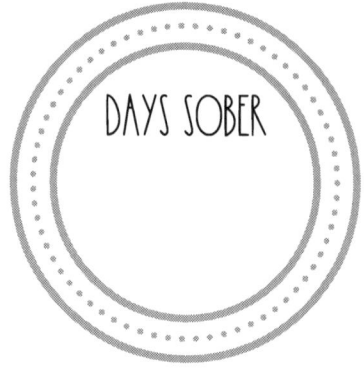

> Our greatest glory is not in never failing, but in rising up every time we fail. R.W. Emerson

TODAY I FEEL ....

TODAY I'M GRATEFUL FOR

1.

2.

3.

TODAY MY GOALS ARE

....

....

....

my mood today:

(1) (2) (3) (4) (5) (6) (7) (8) (9) (10)

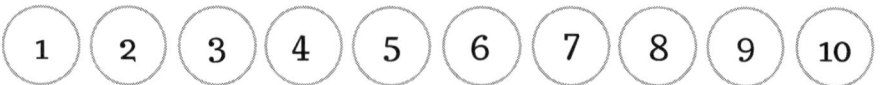

today i will support MY SOBRIETY by doing this ONE thing:

thoughts about today:

date ....

DAYS SOBER

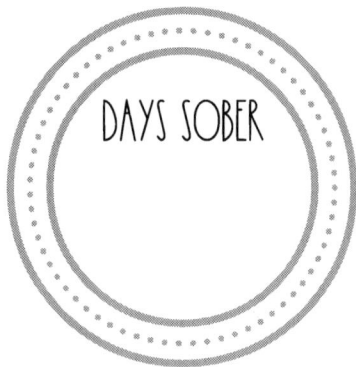

> Strength does
> not come from
> physical capacity.
> It comes from an
> indomitable will. — M. Gandhi

TODAY I FEEL ....

TODAY I'M GRATEFUL FOR

1.

2.

3.

TODAY MY GOALS ARE

....

....

....

my mood today:

(1) (2) (3) (4) (5) (6) (7) (8) (9) (10)

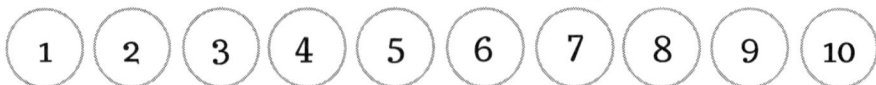

today i will support
MY SOBRIETY
by doing
this ONE thing:

thoughts about today:

date ....

DAYS SOBER

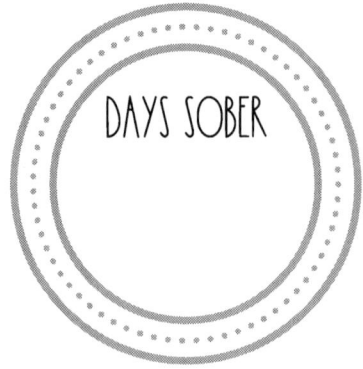

"Life doesn't get easier or more forgiving, we get stronger and more resilient. S. Maraboli

TODAY I FEEL ....

TODAY I'M GRATEFUL FOR

1.

2.

3.

TODAY MY GOALS ARE

....

....

....

my mood today:

(1) (2) (3) (4) (5) (6) (7) (8) (9) (10)

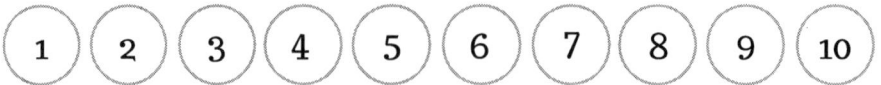

today i will support MY SOBRIETY by doing this ONE thing:

thoughts about today:

date ....

DAYS SOBER

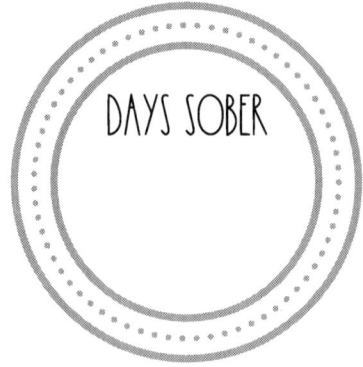

" I avoid looking forward or backward, and try to keep looking upward. " C. Brontë

TODAY I FEEL ....

TODAY I'M GRATEFUL FOR

1.

2.

3.

TODAY MY GOALS ARE

....

....

....

my mood today:

1 2 3 4 5 6 7 8 9 10

today i will support
MY SOBRIETY
by doing
this ONE thing:

thoughts about today:

date ....

DAYS SOBER

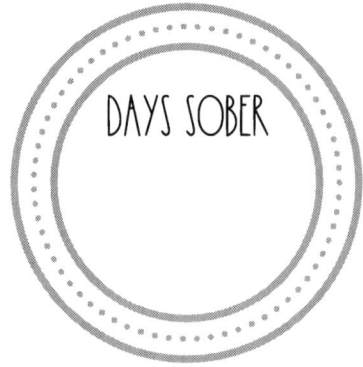

66 The world breaks everyone and afterward many are strong at the broken places. 99 E. Hemingway

TODAY I FEEL ....

TODAY I'M GRATEFUL FOR

1.

2.

3.

TODAY MY GOALS ARE

....

....

....

my mood today:

1 2 3 4 5 6 7 8 9 10

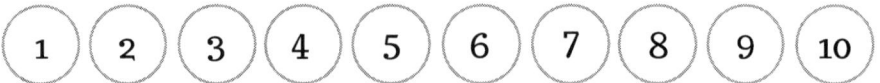

today i will support
MY SOBRIETY
by doing
this ONE thing:

thoughts about today:

date ....

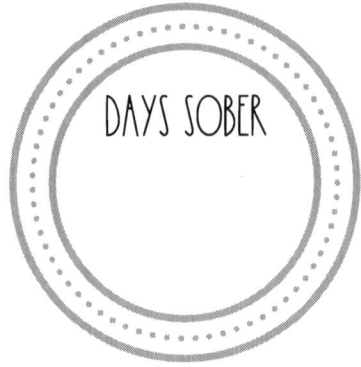

DAYS SOBER

That which does
not kill us makes
us stronger.   F. Nietzsch

TODAY I FEEL ....

TODAY I'M GRATEFUL FOR

1.

2.

3.

TODAY MY GOALS ARE

....

....

....

my mood today:

(1) (2) (3) (4) (5) (6) (7) (8) (9) (10)

today i will support
MY SOBRIETY
by doing
this ONE thing:

thoughts about today:

date ....

DAYS SOBER

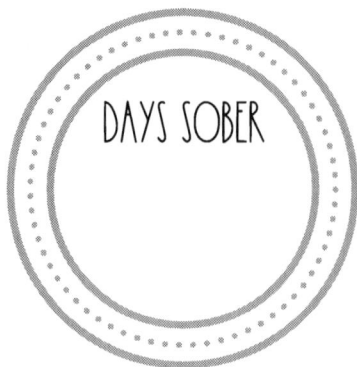

" Change must start
from the individual.
And the individual
must want and
" feel ready to make
such change.   E. Cybulkiewicz

TODAY I FEEL ....

TODAY I'M GRATEFUL FOR

1.

2.

3.

TODAY MY GOALS ARE

....

....

....

my mood today:

(1) (2) (3) (4) (5) (6) (7) (8) (9) (10)

today i will support
MY SOBRIETY
by doing
this ONE thing:

thoughts about today:

date ....

DAYS SOBER

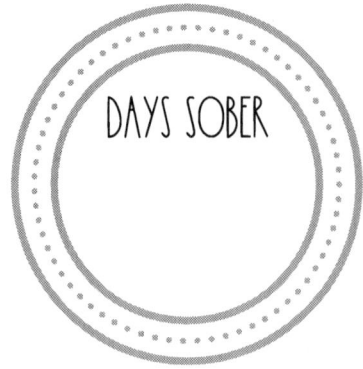

"
Rising from the
ashes, I am born
again, powerful,
exultant, majestic
through all the
pain.   S. Perry
"

TODAY I FEEL ....

TODAY I'M GRATEFUL FOR

1.

2.

3.

TODAY MY GOALS ARE

....

....

....

my mood today:

(1) (2) (3) (4) (5) (6) (7) (8) (9) (10)

today i will support
MY SOBRIETY
by doing
this ONE thing:

thoughts about today:

date ....

DAYS SOBER

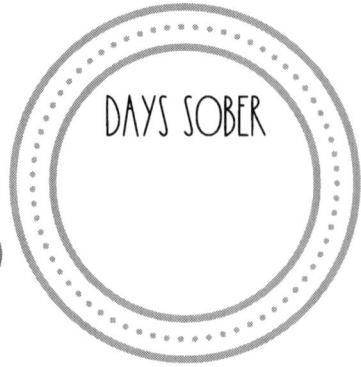

> Anyone can give up; it is the easiest thing in the world to do. But to hold it together when everyone would expect you to fall apart, now that is true strength.   C. Bradford

TODAY I FEEL ....

TODAY I'M GRATEFUL FOR

1.

2.

3.

TODAY MY GOALS ARE

....

....

....

my mood today:

1 2 3 4 5 6 7 8 9 10

today i will support
MY SOBRIETY
by doing
this ONE thing:

thoughts about today:

date ....

DAYS SOBER

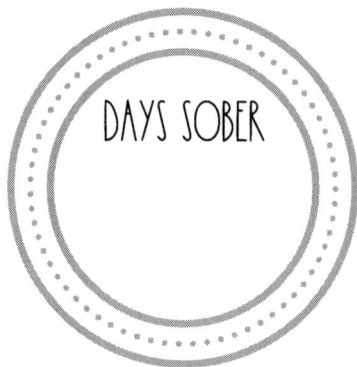

> Courage is
> resistance to fear,
> mastery of fear -
> not absence of
> fear.   M. Twain

TODAY I FEEL ....

TODAY I'M GRATEFUL FOR

1.

2.

3.

TODAY MY GOALS ARE

....

....

....

my mood today:

(1) (2) (3) (4) (5) (6) (7) (8) (9) (10)

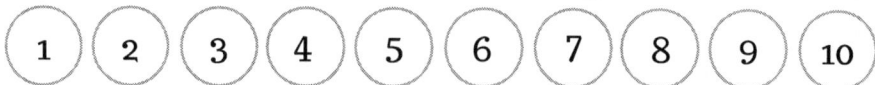

today i will support
MY SOBRIETY
by doing
this ONE thing

thoughts about today:

date ....

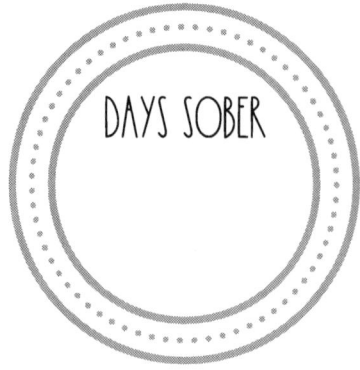
DAYS SOBER

No matter how dark the night may get, your light will never burn out. J. LeBlanc

TODAY I FEEL ....

TODAY I'M GRATEFUL FOR

1.

2.

3.

TODAY MY GOALS ARE

....

....

....

my mood today:

(1) (2) (3) (4) (5) (6) (7) (8) (9) (10)

today i will support MY SOBRIETY *by doing* this ONE thing:

thoughts about today:

date ....

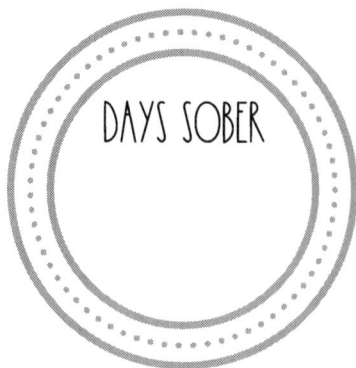

> "If we are facing in the right direction, all we have to do is keep on walking." Zen proverb

TODAY I FEEL ....

TODAY I'M GRATEFUL FOR

1.

2.

3.

TODAY MY GOALS ARE

....

....

....

my mood today:

(1) (2) (3) (4) (5) (6) (7) (8) (9) (10)

today i will support MY SOBRIETY *by doing* this ONE thing:

thoughts about today:

date ....

DAYS SOBER

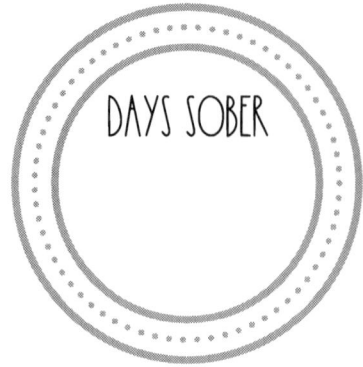

" Either you run
the day, or the
day runs you. J. Rohn

TODAY I FEEL ....

TODAY I'M GRATEFUL FOR

1.

2.

3.

TODAY MY GOALS ARE

....

....

....

my mood today:

(1) (2) (3) (4) (5) (6) (7) (8) (9) (10)

today i will support
MY SOBRIETY
by doing
this ONE thing:

thoughts about today:

date ....

DAYS SOBER

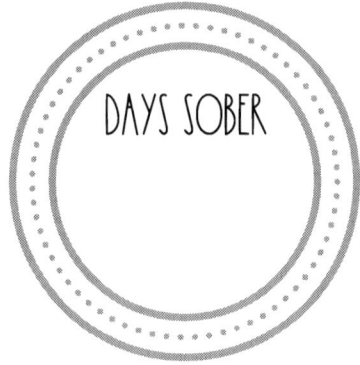

" People often say
that motivation
doesn't last. Neither
does bathing. That's
" why we recommend
it daily.   Z. Ziglar

TODAY I FEEL ....

TODAY I'M GRATEFUL FOR

1.

2.

3.

TODAY MY GOALS ARE

....

....

....

my mood today:

(1) (2) (3) (4) (5) (6) (7) (8) (9) (10)

today i will support
MY SOBRIETY
by doing
this ONE thing:

thoughts about today:

date _____

DAYS SOBER

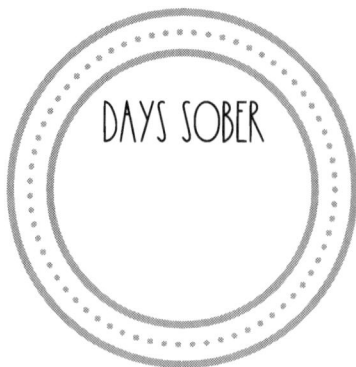

" No other road,
no other way,
no day but
today.   J. Larson

TODAY I FEEL _____

TODAY I'M GRATEFUL FOR

1.

2.

3.

TODAY MY GOALS ARE

_____

_____

_____

my mood today:

(1) (2) (3) (4) (5) (6) (7) (8) (9) (10)

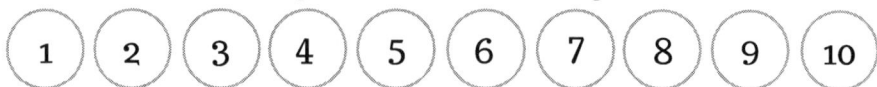

today i will support
MY SOBRIETY
by doing
this ONE thing

thoughts about today:

$date$ ....

DAYS SOBER

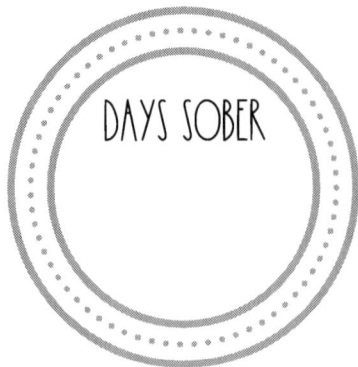

> Don't judge
> each day by the
> harvest you
> reap but by the
> seeds that you
> plant. R.L. Stevenson

TODAY I FEEL ....

TODAY I'M GRATEFUL FOR

1.

2.

3.

TODAY MY GOALS ARE

....

....

....

my mood today:

(1) (2) (3) (4) (5) (6) (7) (8) (9) (10)

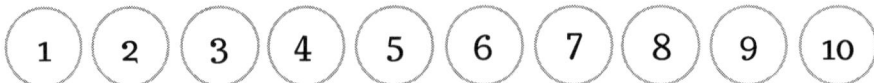

today i will support
MY SOBRIETY
by doing
this ONE thing:

thoughts about today:

_____
_____
_____
_____
_____
_____
_____
_____
_____

date ....

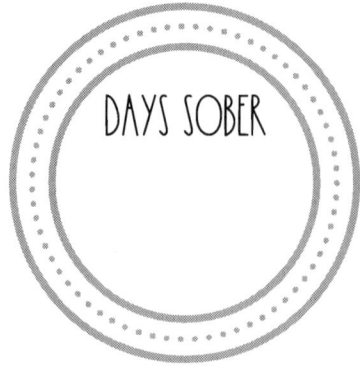

DAYS SOBER

> As human beings,
> our greatness lies
> not so much in being
> able to remake the
> world... as in being
> able to remake
> ourselves.   M. Gandhi

TODAY I FEEL ....

TODAY I'M GRATEFUL FOR

1.

2.

3.

TODAY MY GOALS ARE

....

....

....

my mood today:

(1) (2) (3) (4) (5) (6) (7) (8) (9) (10)

today i will support
MY SOBRIETY
by doing
this ONE thing:

thoughts about today:

date ....

DAYS SOBER

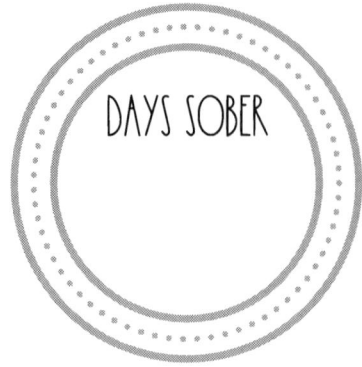

" The man who makes no mistakes does not usually make anything. " B. W.C. Magee

TODAY I FEEL ....

TODAY I'M GRATEFUL FOR

1.

2.

3.

TODAY MY GOALS ARE

....

....

....

my mood today:

1 2 3 4 5 6 7 8 9 10

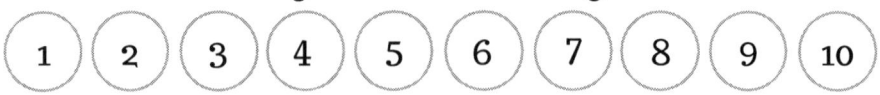

today i will support
MY SOBRIETY
by doing
this ONE thing:

thoughts about today:

date ....

DAYS SOBER

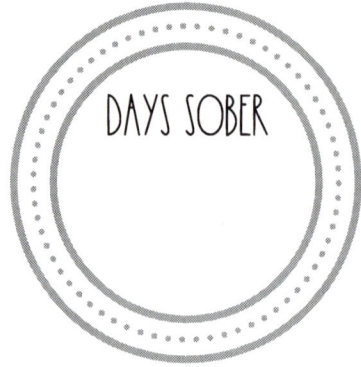

" Recovery is not a race. You don't have to feel guilty if it takes you longer than you thought it would. " Unknown

TODAY I FEEL ....

TODAY I'M GRATEFUL FOR

1.

2.

3.

TODAY MY GOALS ARE

....

....

....

my mood today:

(1) (2) (3) (4) (5) (6) (7) (8) (9) (10)

today i will support MY SOBRIETY *by doing* this ONE thing:

thoughts about today:

date

_____

DAYS SOBER

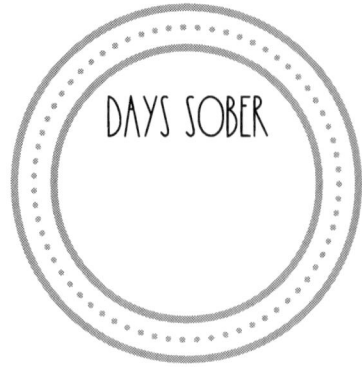

"" Addiction brings
apathy. Break the
apathy, and you
break the
addiction. — M. Wodzak

TODAY I FEEL

_____

TODAY I'M GRATEFUL FOR

1.

2.

3.

TODAY MY GOALS ARE

_____

_____

_____

my mood today:

(1) (2) (3) (4) (5) (6) (7) (8) (9) (10)

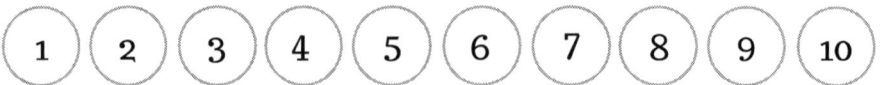

today i will support
MY SOBRIETY
by doing
this ONE thing:

thoughts about today:

date ....

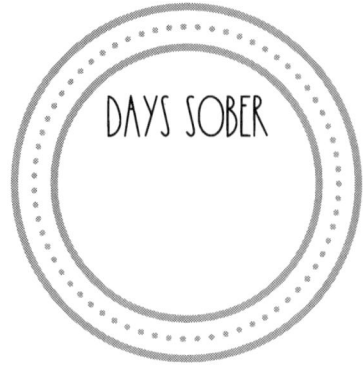

Remember just
because you hit
bottom doesn't
mean you have to
stay there. R. Downey Jr.

TODAY I FEEL ....

TODAY I'M GRATEFUL FOR

1.

2.

3.

TODAY MY GOALS ARE

....

....

....

my mood today:

(1) (2) (3) (4) (5) (6) (7) (8) (9) (10)

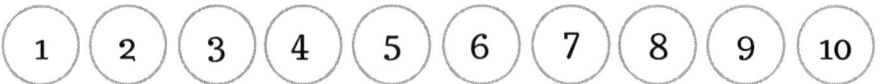

today i will support
MY SOBRIETY
by doing
this ONE thing:

thoughts about today:

date ....

DAYS SOBER

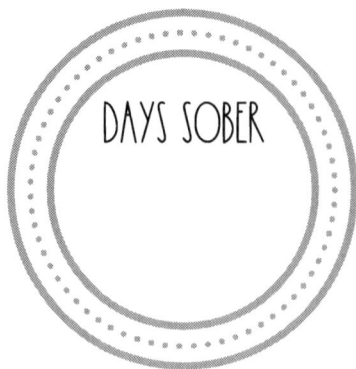

> Recovery is something you have to work on every single day, and it's something that doesn't get a day off.   D Lovato

TODAY I FEEL ....

TODAY I'M GRATEFUL FOR

1.

2.

3.

TODAY MY GOALS ARE

....

....

....

my mood today:

(1) (2) (3) (4) (5) (6) (7) (8) (9) (10)

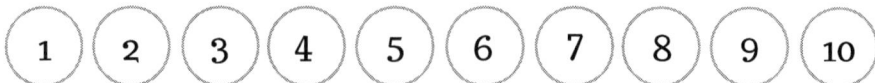

today i will support
MY SOBRIETY
by doing
this ONE thing:

thoughts about today:

date ....

DAYS SOBER

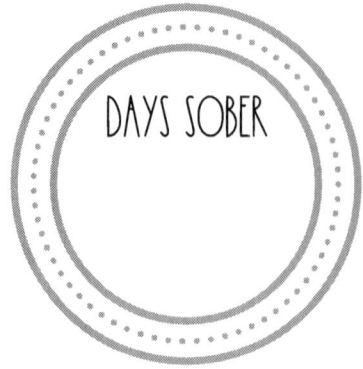

"
We need never be
hopeless because
we can never be
irreparably
broken.   J. Green
"

TODAY I FEEL ....

TODAY I'M GRATEFUL FOR

1.

2.

3.

TODAY MY GOALS ARE

....

....

....

my mood today:

(1) (2) (3) (4) (5) (6) (7) (8) (9) (10)

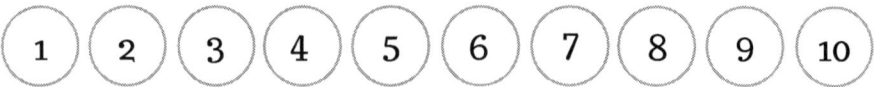

today i will support
MY SOBRIETY
by doing
this ONE thing:

thoughts about today:

date ....

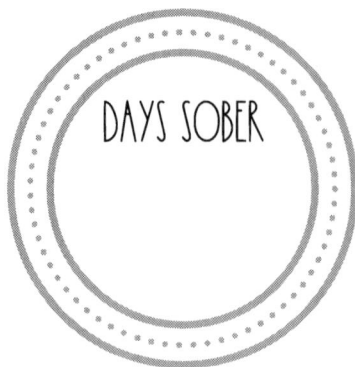

> You have brains in your head. You have feet in your shoes. You can steer yourself any direction you choose. — Dr. Seuss

TODAY I FEEL ....

TODAY I'M GRATEFUL FOR

1.

2.

3.

TODAY MY GOALS ARE

....

....

....

my mood today:

(1) (2) (3) (4) (5) (6) (7) (8) (9) (10)

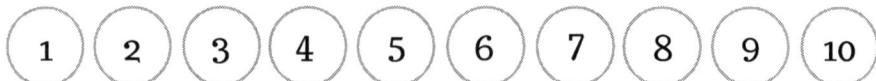

today i will support MY SOBRIETY by doing this ONE thing:

thoughts about today:

_____
_____
_____
_____
_____
_____
_____
_____
_____

date ....

DAYS SOBER

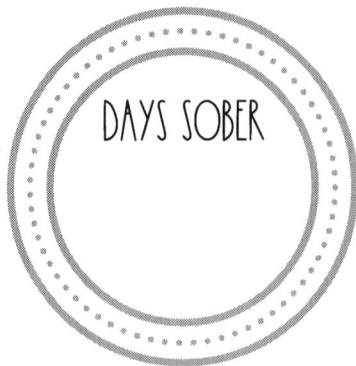

" The diamond cannot be polished without friction, nor the person perfected without trials. " Chinese proverb

TODAY I FEEL ....

TODAY I'M GRATEFUL FOR

1.

2.

3.

TODAY MY GOALS ARE

....

....

....

my mood today:

(1) (2) (3) (4) (5) (6) (7) (8) (9) (10)

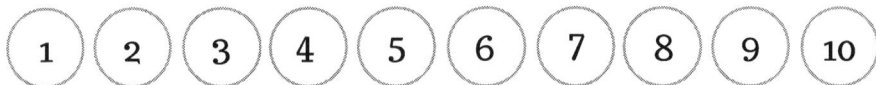

today i will support MY SOBRIETY *by doing* this ONE thing:

thoughts about today:

date ....

DAYS SOBER

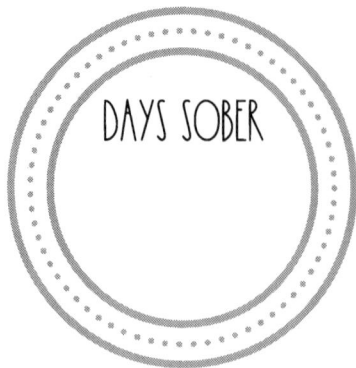

66 You have to
break down
before you can
break through. 99 M. Ferguson

TODAY I FEEL ....

TODAY I'M GRATEFUL FOR

1.

2.

3.

TODAY MY GOALS ARE

....

....

....

my mood today:

(1) (2) (3) (4) (5) (6) (7) (8) (9) (10)

today i will support
MY SOBRIETY
by doing
this ONE thing:

thoughts about today:

date ....

DAYS SOBER

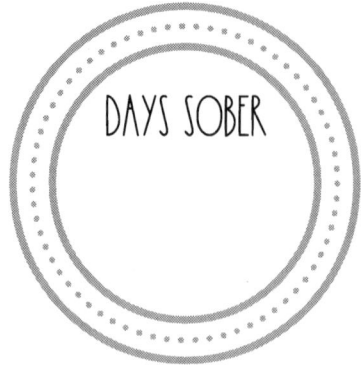

" Rock bottom
became the solid
foundation on
which I rebuilt
my life.   J.K. Rowling

TODAY I FEEL ....

TODAY I'M GRATEFUL FOR

1.

2.

3.

TODAY MY GOALS ARE

....

....

....

my mood today:

(1) (2) (3) (4) (5) (6) (7) (8) (9) (10)

today i will support
MY SOBRIETY
by doing
this ONE thing

thoughts about today:

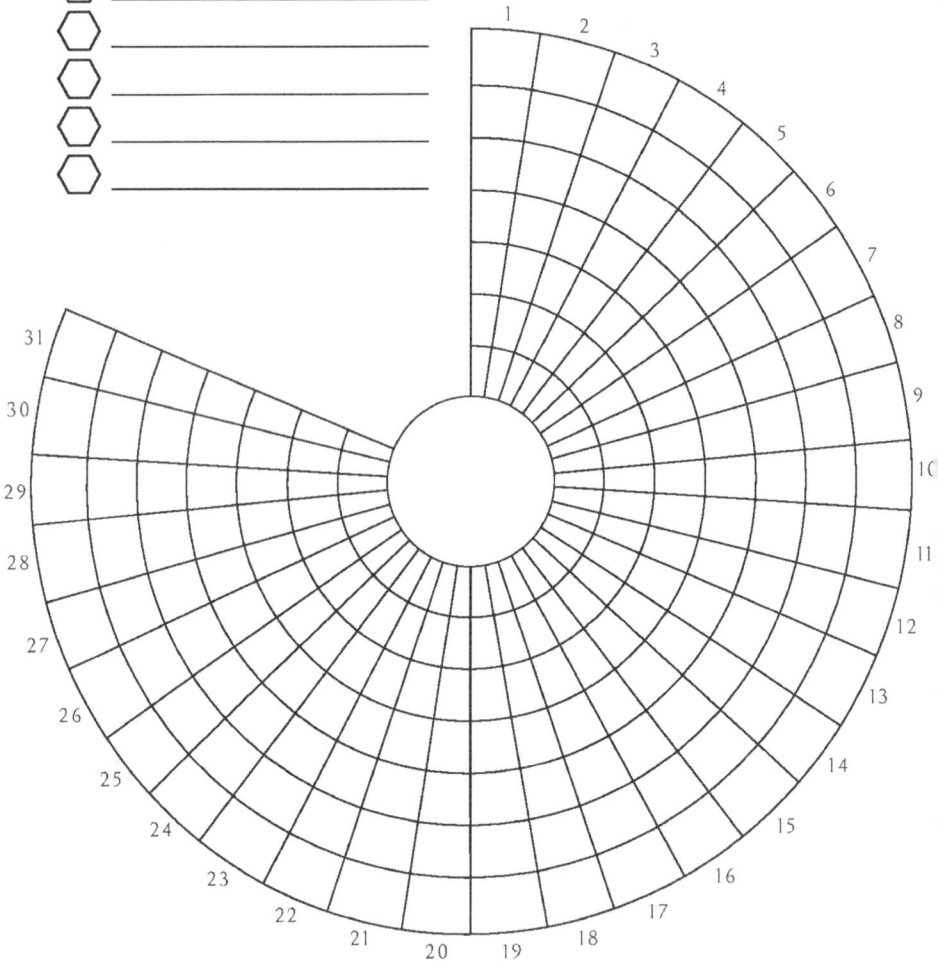

MY MONTH *at a glance*

HABIT TRACKER

MONTH: _____

COLOR · · · ESSENTIAL HABITS

⬡ _____
⬡ _____
⬡ _____
⬡ _____
⬡ _____
⬡ _____
⬡ _____

1 2 3 4 5 6 7 8 9 10 11 12 13 14 15 16 17 18 19 20 21 22 23 24 25 26 27 28 29 30 31

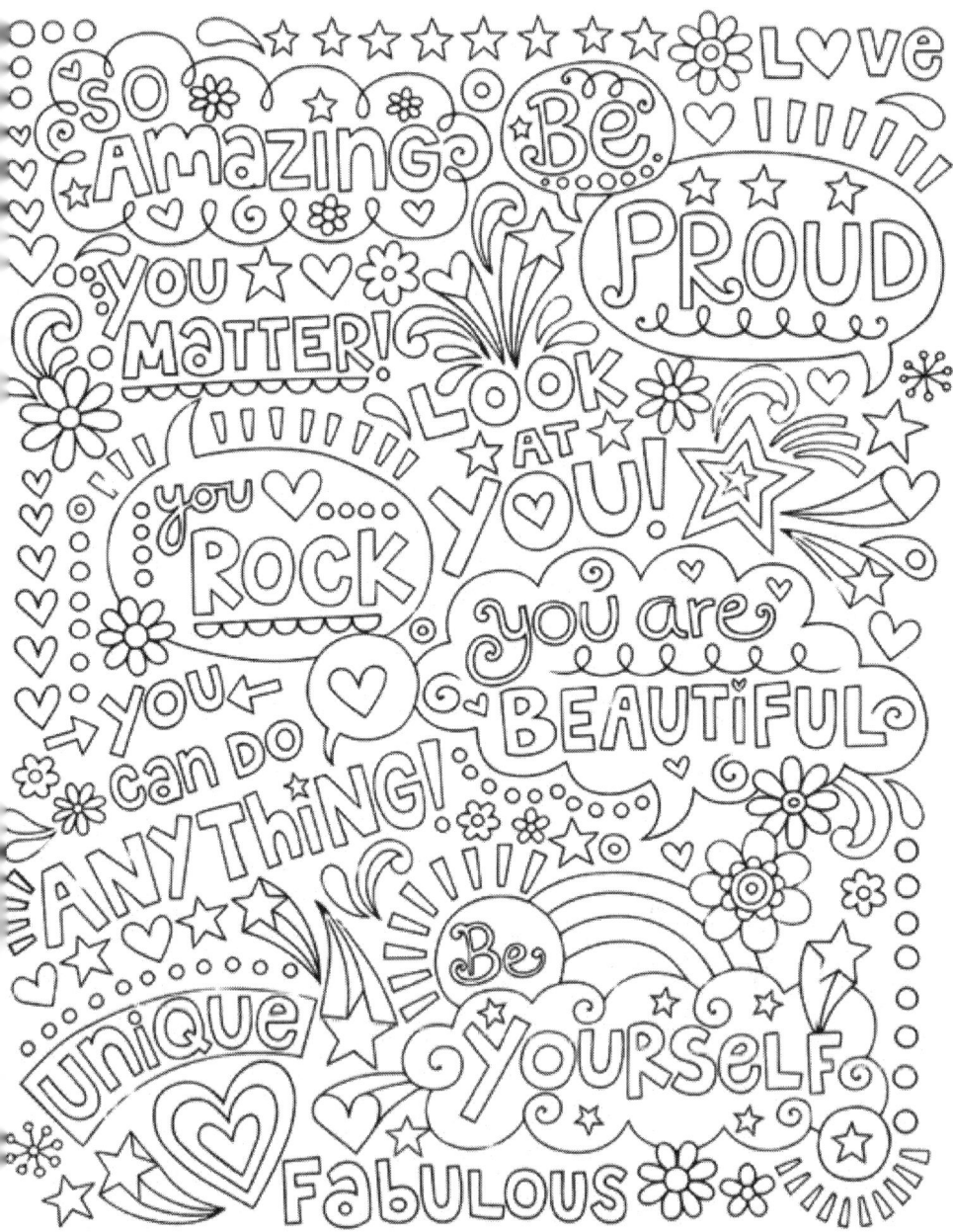

So Amazing!
You Matter!
Be
LOVE
PROUD
You Rock
LOOK AT YOU!
You can do ANYTHING!
You are BEAUTIFUL
Unique
Be Yourself
Fabulous

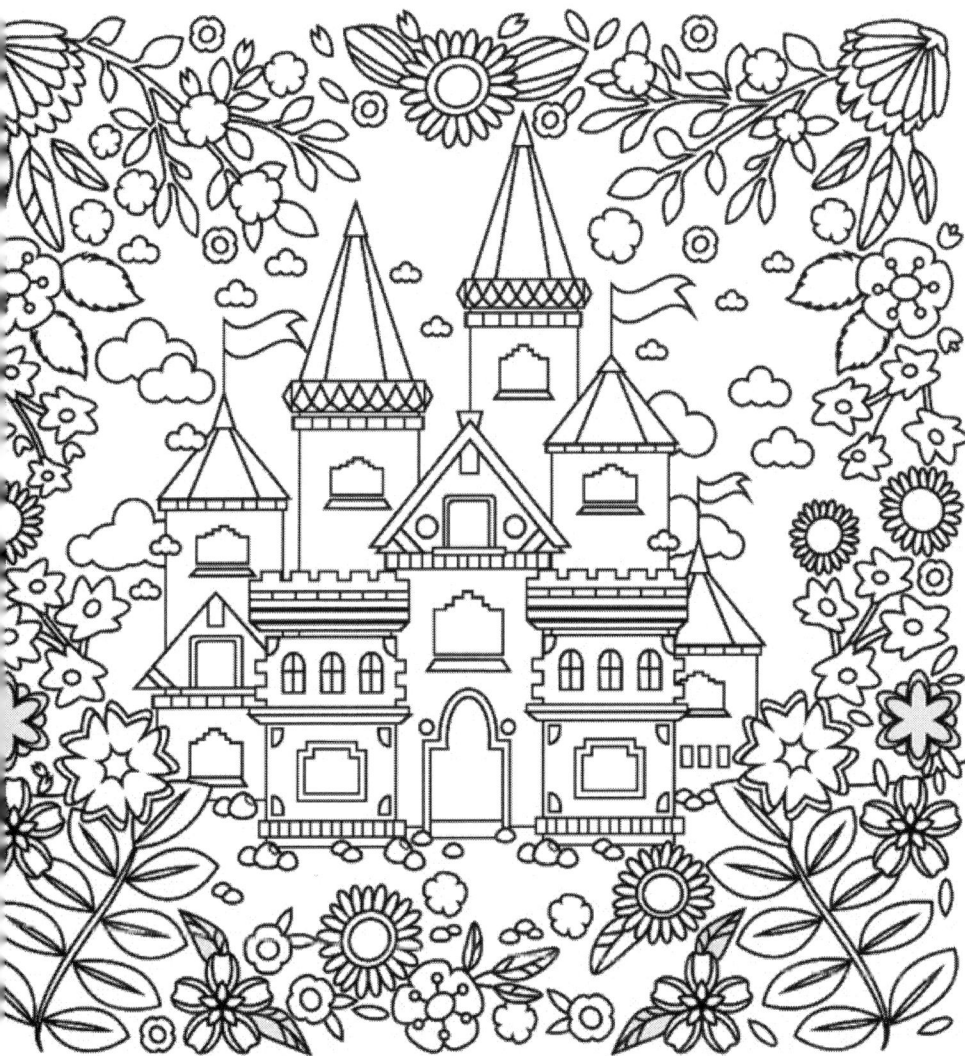

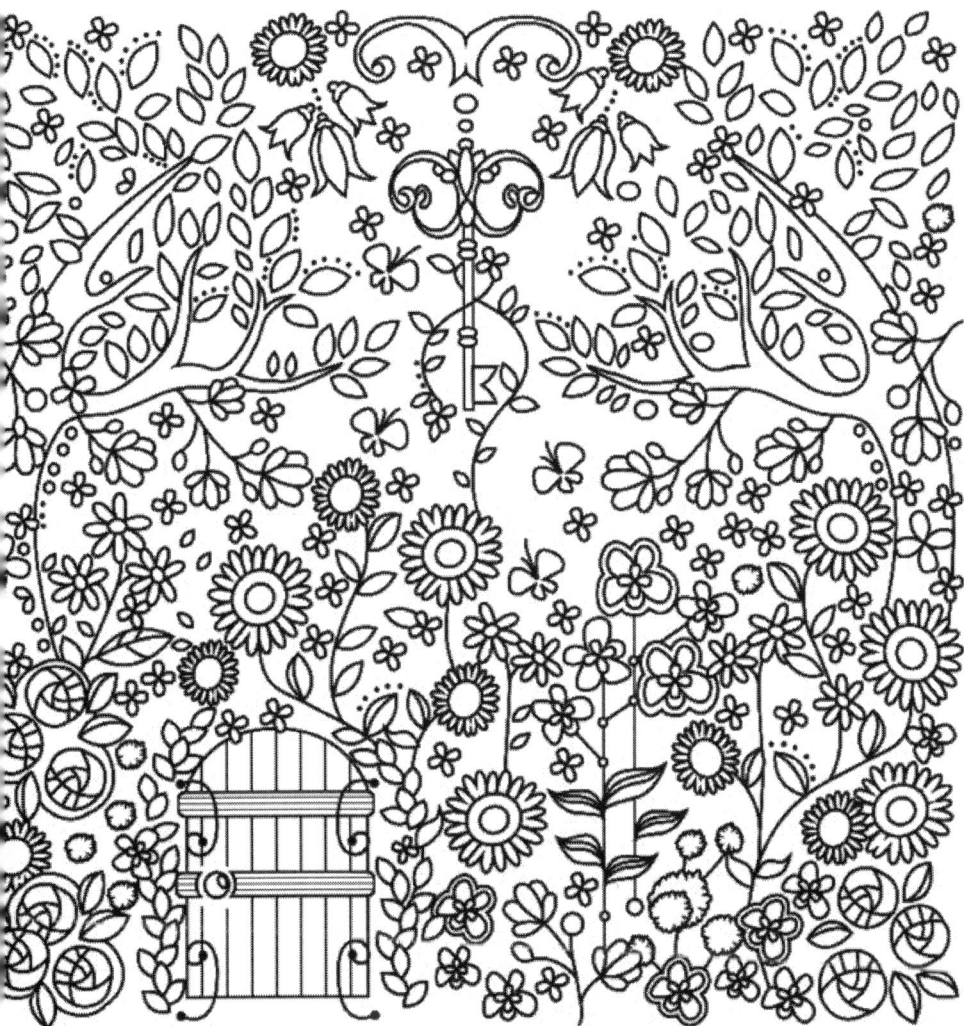

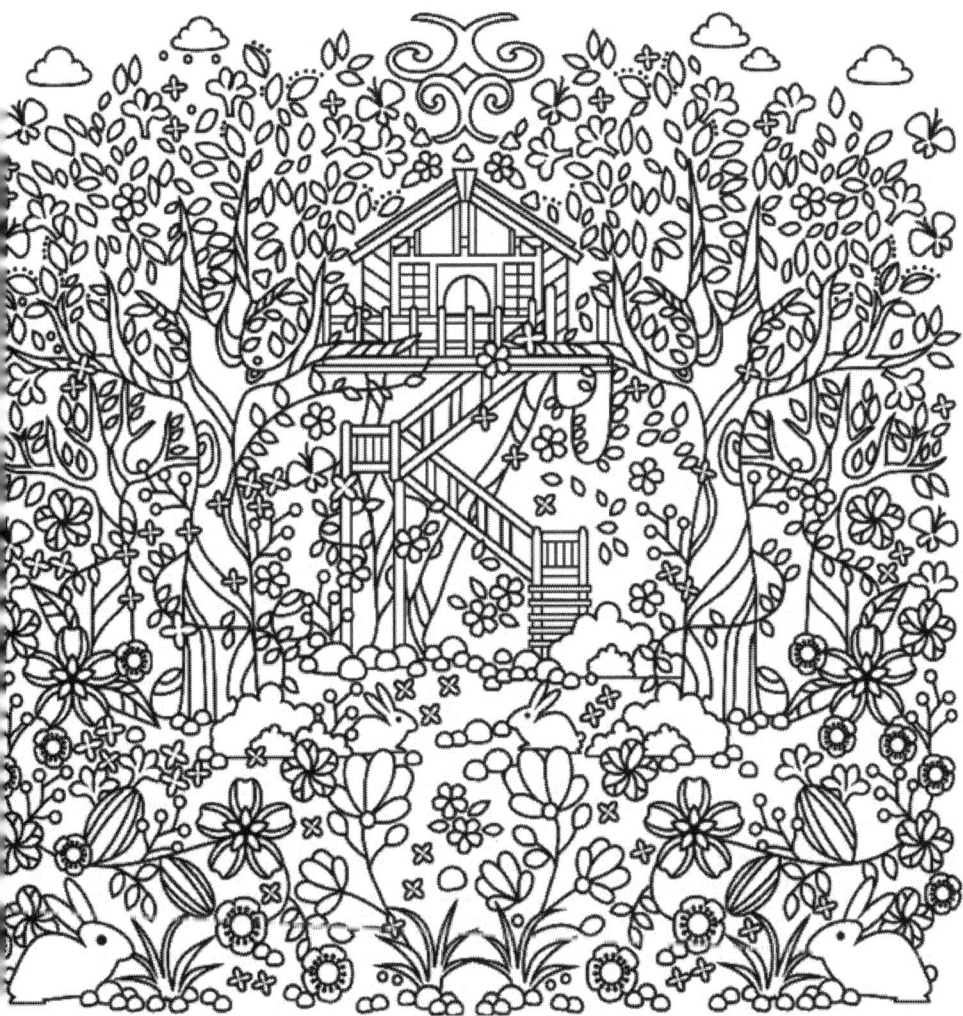

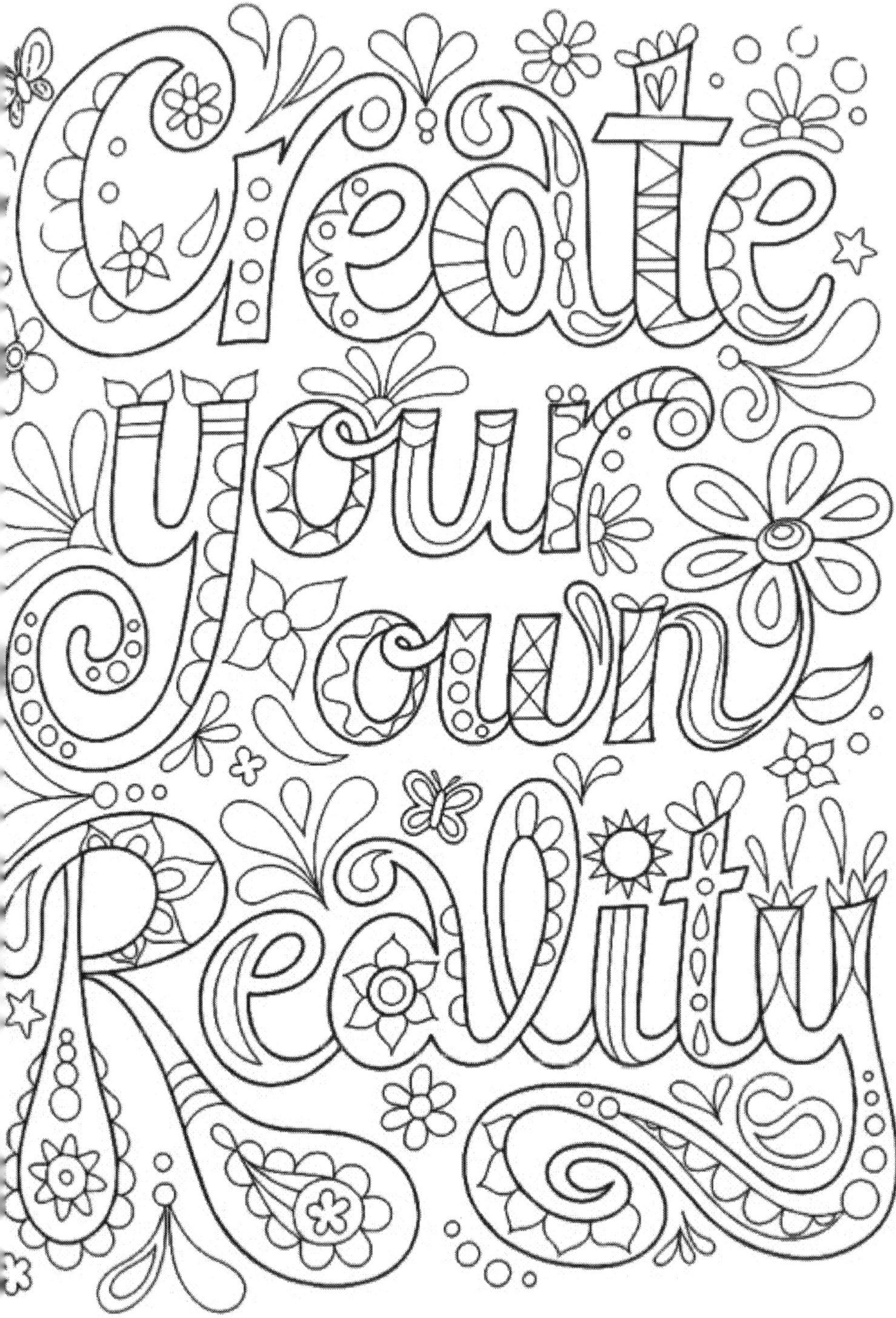
Create your own Reality

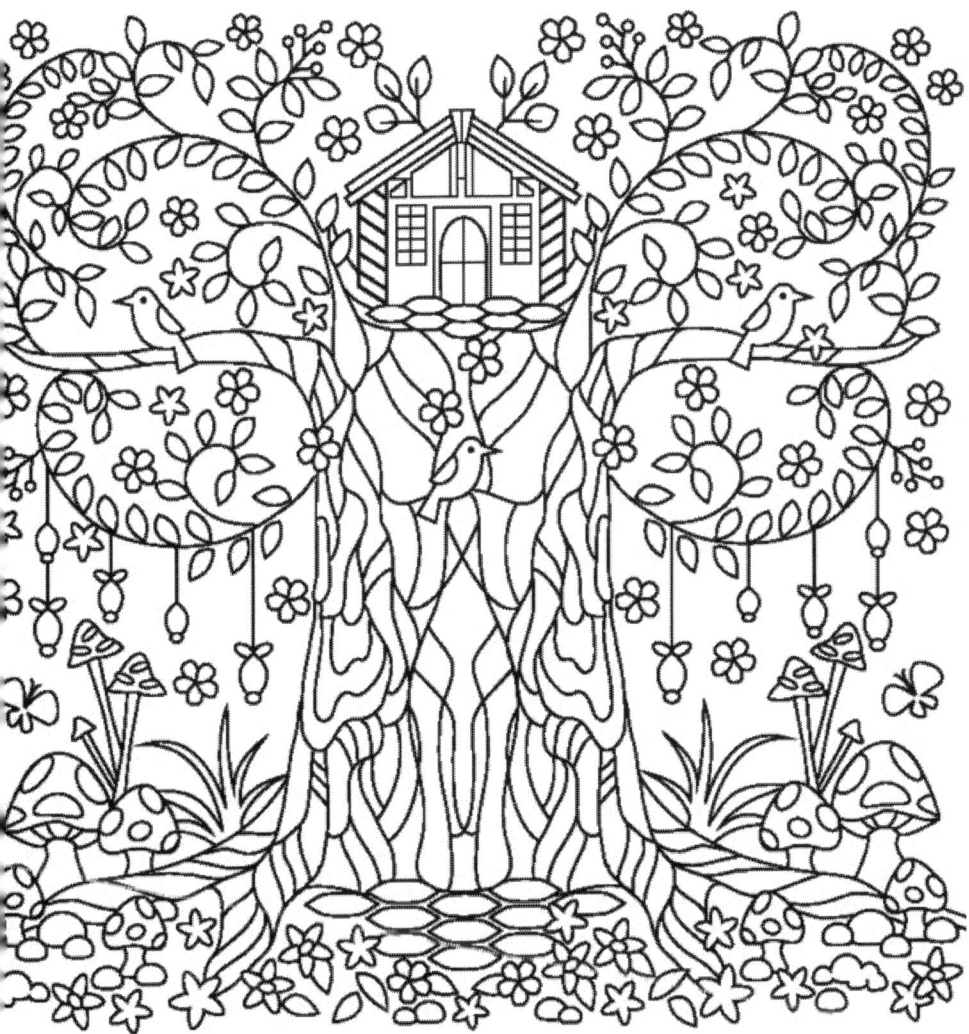

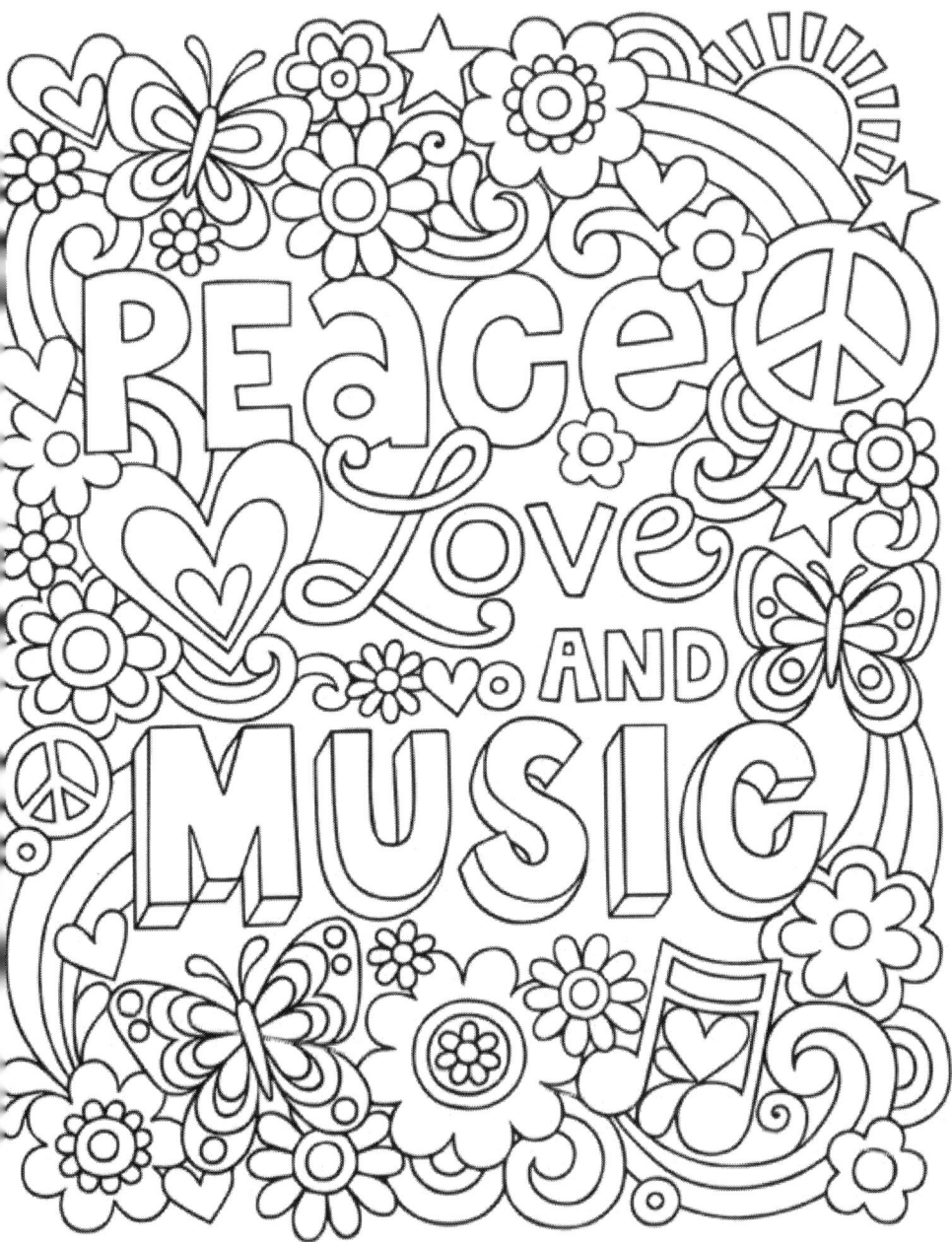

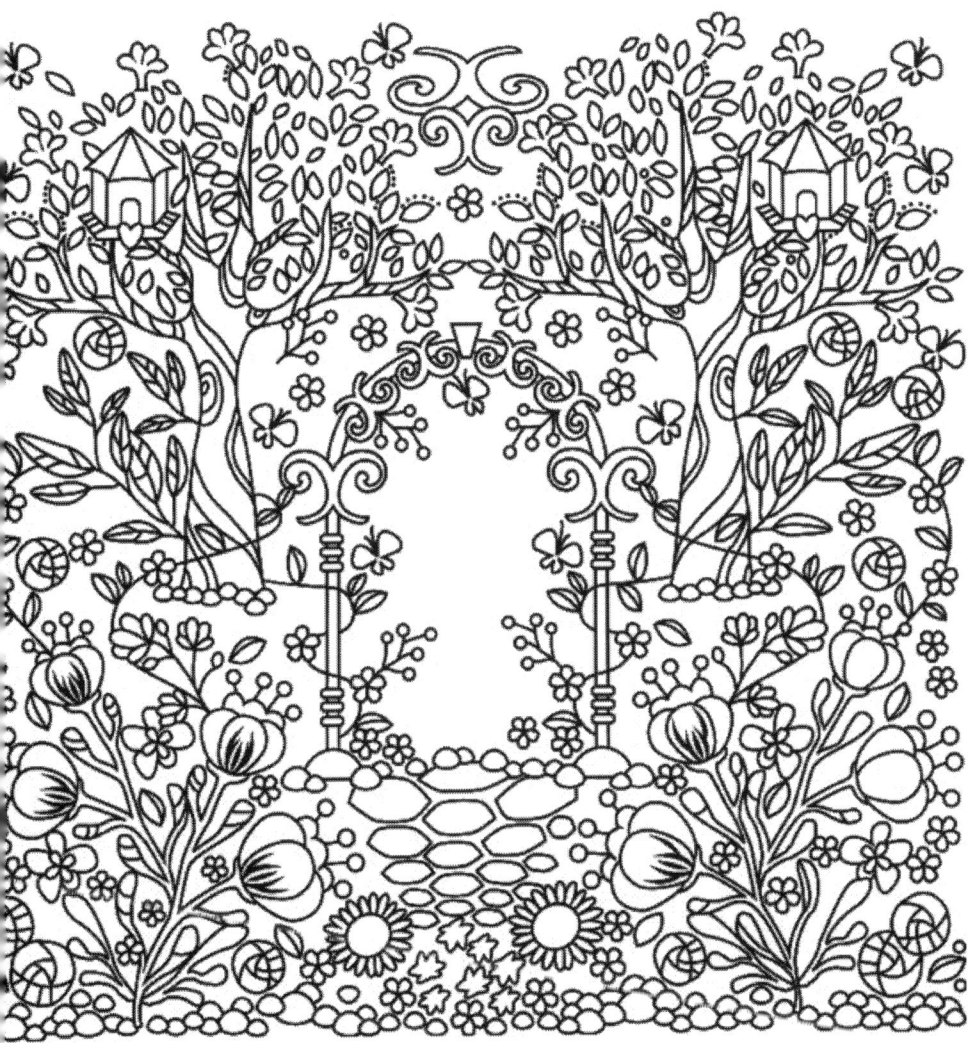

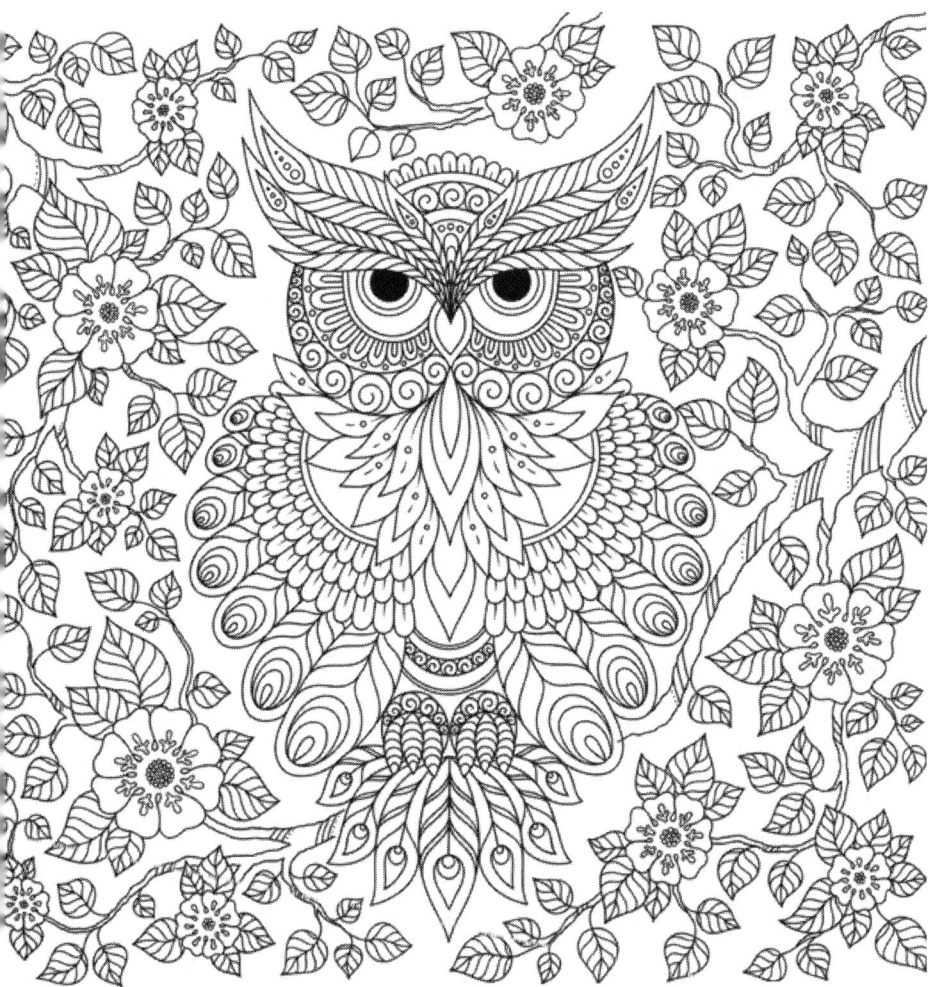

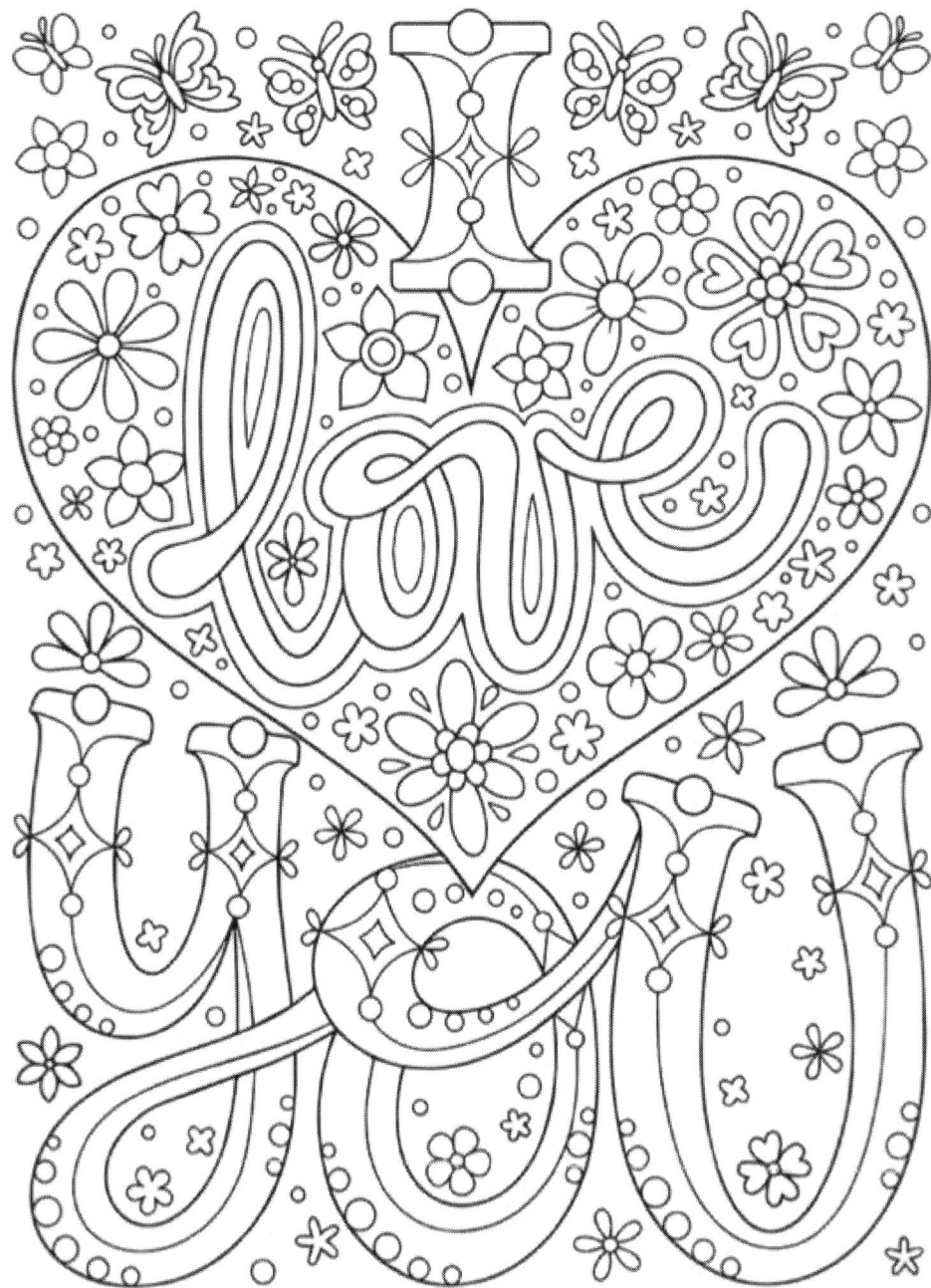

Manufactured by Amazon.ca
Bolton, ON

29613180R00081